Content

About acne

Acne is a common skin condition that affects most people at some point. It causes spots, oily skin and sometimes skin that's hot or painful to touch.

Acne most commonly develops on the:

• face – this affects almost everyone with acne

• back – this affects more than half of people with acne

• chest – this affects about 15% of people with acne

Types of spots

There are 6 main types of spot caused by acne:

• blackheads – small black or yellowish bumps that develop on the skin; they're not filled with dirt, but are black because the inner lining of the hair follicle produces pigmentation (colouring)

• whiteheads – have a similar appearance to blackheads, but may be firmer and won't empty when squeezed

• papules – small red bumps that may feel tender or sore

• pustules – similar to papules, but have a white tip in the centre, caused by a build-up of pus

• nodules – large hard lumps that build up beneath the surface of the skin and can be painful

• cysts – the most severe type of spot caused by acne; they're large pus-filled lumps that look similar to boils and carry the greatest risk of causing permanent scarring

What can I do if I have acne?

The self-help techniques below may be useful:

• Don't wash affected areas of skin more than twice a day. Frequent washing can irritate the skin and make symptoms worse

• Wash the affected area with a mild soap or cleanser and lukewarm water. Very hot or cold water can make acne worse

• Don't try to "clean out" blackheads or squeeze spots. This can make them worse and cause permanent scarring

• Avoid using too much make-up and cosmetics. Use water-based products that are described as non-comedogenic (this means the product is less likely to block the pores in your skin)

• Completely remove make-up before going to bed

• If dry skin is a problem, use a fragrance-free, water-based emollient

• Regular exercise can't improve your acne, but it can boost your mood and improve your self-esteem. Shower as soon as possible once you finish exercising, as sweat can irritate your acne

• Wash your hair regularly and try to avoid letting your hair fall across your face

Although acne can't be cured, it can be controlled with treatment. Several creams, lotions and gels for treating spots are available at pharmacies. If you develop acne, it's a good idea to speak to your pharmacist for advice.

Treatments can take up to 3 months to work, so don't expect results overnight. Once they do start to work, the results are usually good.

Causes of acne

Acne is caused when tiny holes in the skin, known as hair follicles, become blocked.

Sebaceous glands are tiny glands found near the surface of your skin. The glands are attached to hair follicles, which are small holes in your skin that an individual hair grows out of.

Sebaceous glands lubricate the hair and the skin to stop it drying out. They do this by producing an oily substance called sebum.

In acne, the glands begin to produce too much sebum. The excess sebum mixes with dead skin cells and both substances form a plug in the follicle.

If the plugged follicle is close to the surface of the skin, it bulges outwards, creating a whitehead. Alternatively, the plugged follicle can be open to the skin, creating a blackhead.

Normally harmless bacteria that live on the skin can then contaminate and infect the plugged follicles, causing papules, pustules, nodules or cysts.

Testosterone

Teenage acne is thought to be triggered by increased levels of a hormone called testosterone, which occurs during puberty. The hormone plays an important role in stimulating the growth and development of the penis and testicles in boys, and maintaining muscle and bone strength in girls.

The sebaceous glands are particularly sensitive to hormones. It's thought that increased levels of testosterone cause the glands to produce much more sebum than the skin needs.

Acne in families

Acne can run in families. If your parents had acne, it's likely that you'll also develop it.

One study has found that if both your parents had acne, you're more likely to get more severe acne at an early age. It also found that if one or both of your parents had adult acne, you're more likely to get adult acne too.

Acne in women

More than 80% of cases of adult acne occur in women. It's thought that many cases of adult acne are caused by the changes in hormone levels that many women have at certain times.

These times include:

• periods – some women have a flare-up of acne just before their period

• pregnancy – many women have symptoms of acne at this time, usually during the first 3 months of their pregnancy

• polycystic ovary syndrome – a common condition that can cause acne, weight gain and the formation of small cysts inside the ovary

Other triggers

Other possible triggers of an acne flare-up include:

• some cosmetic products – however, this is less common as most products are now tested, so they don't cause spots (non-comedogenic)

• certain medications – such as steroid medications, lithium (used to treat depression and bipolar disorder) and some anti-epileptic drugs (used to treat epilepsy)

• regularly wearing items that place pressure on an affected area of skin, such as a headband or backpack

• smoking – which can contribute to acne in older people

Acne myths

Despite being one of the most widespread skin conditions, acne is also one of the most poorly understood. There are many myths and misconceptions about it:

"Acne is caused by a poor diet"

So far, research hasn't found any foods that cause acne. Eating a healthy, balanced diet is recommended because it's good for your heart and your health in general.

"Acne is caused by having dirty skin and poor hygiene"

Most of the biological reactions that trigger acne occur beneath the skin, not on the surface, so the cleanliness of your skin has no effect on your acne. Washing your face more than twice a day could just aggravate your skin.

"Squeezing blackheads, whiteheads and spots is the best way to get rid of acne"

This could actually make symptoms worse and may leave you with scarring.

"Sexual activity can influence acne"

Having sex or masturbating won't make acne any better or worse.

"Sunbathing, sunbeds and sunlamps help improve the symptoms of acne"

There's no conclusive evidence that prolonged exposure to sunlight or using sunbeds or sunlamps can improve acne.

Many medications used to treat acne can make your skin more sensitive to light, so exposure could cause painful damage to your skin, and also increase your risk of skin cancer.

"Acne is infectious"

You can't pass acne on to other people.

Diagnosing acne

Your pharmacist can diagnose acne by looking at your skin. This involves examining your face and possibly your chest and back for different types of spot, such as blackheads or sore, red nodules.

How many spots you have and how painful and inflamed they are will help determine how severe your acne is. This is important in planning your treatment.

4 grades can be used to measure the severity of acne:

• grade 1 (mild) – acne is mostly confined to whiteheads and blackheads, with just a few papules and pustules

• grade 2 (moderate) – there are multiple papules and pustules, which are mostly confined to the face

• grade 3 (moderately severe) – there's a large number of papules and pustules, as well as the occasional inflamed nodule, and the back and chest are also affected by acne

• grade 4 (severe) – there's a large number of large, painful pustules and nodules

Acne in women

If acne suddenly starts in adult women, it can be a sign of a hormonal imbalance, especially if it's accompanied by other symptoms such as:

• excessive body hair (hirsutism)

• irregular or light periods

The most common cause of hormonal imbalances in women is polycystic ovary syndrome (PCOS). PCOS can be diagnosed using a combination of ultrasound scans and blood tests.

Treating acne

Treatment for acne depends on how severe it is. It can take several months of treatment before acne symptoms improve.

The various treatments for acne are outlined below.

If you just have a few blackheads, whiteheads and spots, you should be able to treat them successfully with over-the-counter gels or creams (topical treatments) that contain benzoyl peroxide.

Treatments from your GP

See your GP if your acne is more widespread, as you probably need prescription medication. For example, if:

• you have a large number of papules and pustules

• over-the-counter medication hasn't worked

Prescription medications that can be used to treat acne include:

• topical retinoids

• topical antibiotics

• azelaic acid

- antibiotic tablets

- in women, the combined oral contraceptive pill

- isotretinoin tablets

If you have severe acne, your GP can refer you to an expert in treating skin conditions (dermatologist). For example, if you have:

- a large number of papules and pustules on your chest and back, as well as your face

- painful nodules

A combination of antibiotic tablets and topical treatments is usually the first treatment option for severe acne. If this doesn't work, a medication called isotretinoin may be prescribed.

Hormonal therapies or the combined oral contraceptive pill can also be effective in women who have acne. However, the progestogen-only pill or contraceptive implant can sometimes make acne worse.

Many of these treatments can take 2 to 3 months before they start to work. It's important to be patient and persist with a recommended treatment, even if there's no immediate effect.

Topical treatments (gels, creams and lotions)

Benzoyl peroxide

Benzoyl peroxide works as an antiseptic to reduce the number of bacteria on the surface of the skin. It also helps to reduce the number of whiteheads and blackheads, and has an anti-inflammatory effect.

Benzoyl peroxide is usually available as a cream or gel. It's used either once or twice a day. It should be applied 20 minutes after washing to all of the parts of your face affected by acne.

It should be used sparingly, as too much can irritate your skin. It also makes your face more sensitive to sunlight, so avoid too much sun and ultraviolet (UV) light, or wear sun cream.

Benzoyl peroxide can have a bleaching effect, so avoid getting it on your hair or clothes.

Common side effects of benzoyl peroxide include:

• dry and tense skin

• a burning, itching or stinging sensation

• some redness and peeling of the skin

Side effects are usually mild and should pass once the treatment has finished.

Most people need a 6 week course of treatment to clear most or all of their acne. You may be advised to continue treatment less frequently to prevent acne returning.

Topical retinoids

Topical retinoids work by removing dead skin cells from the surface of the skin (exfoliating) which helps to prevent them building up within hair follicles.

Tretinoin and adapalene are topical retinoids used to treat acne. They're available in a gel or cream and are usually applied once a day before you go to bed.

Apply to all the parts of your face affected by acne 20 minutes after washing your face.

It's important to apply topical retinoids sparingly and avoid excessive exposure to sunlight and UV.

Topical retinoids aren't suitable for use during pregnancy, as there's a risk they might cause birth defects.

The most common side effects of topical retinoids are mild irritation and stinging of the skin.

A 6 week course is usually required, but you may be advised to continue using the medication less frequently after this.

Topical antibiotics

Topical antibiotics help kill the bacteria on the skin that can infect plugged hair follicles. They're available as a lotion or gel that is applied once or twice a day.

A 6 to 8 week course is usually recommended. After this, treatment is usually stopped, as there's a risk that the bacteria on your face could become resistant to the antibiotics. This could make your acne worse and cause additional infections.

Side effects are uncommon, but can include:

• minor irritation of the skin

• redness and burning of the skin

• peeling of the skin

Azelaic acid

Azelaic acid is often used as an alternative treatment for acne if the side effects of benzoyl peroxide or topical retinoids are particularly irritating or painful.

Azelaic acid works by getting rid of dead skin and killing bacteria. It's available as a cream or gel and is usually applied twice a day (or once a day if your skin is particularly sensitive).

The medication doesn't make your skin sensitive to sunlight, so you don't have to avoid exposure to the sun.

You'll usually need to use azelaic acid for a month before your acne improves.

The side effects of azelaic acid are usually mild and include:

• burning or stinging skin

• itchiness

• dry skin

• redness of the skin

Antibiotic tablets

Antibiotic tablets (oral antibiotics) are usually used in combination with a topical treatment to treat more severe acne.

In most cases, a class of antibiotics called tetracyclines is prescribed, unless you're pregnant or breastfeeding.

Pregnant or breastfeeding women are usually advised to take an antibiotic called erythromycin, which is known to be safer to use.

It usually takes about 6 weeks before you notice an improvement in your acne.

Depending on how well you react to the treatment, a course of oral antibiotics can last 4 to 6 months.

Tetracyclines can make your skin sensitive to sunlight and UV light, and can also make the oral contraceptive pill less effective during the first few weeks of treatment.

You'll need to use an alternative method of contraception, such as condoms, during this time.

Hormonal therapies

Hormonal therapies can often benefit women with acne, especially if the acne flares up around periods or is associated with hormonal conditions such as polycystic ovary syndrome.

If you don't already use it, your GP may recommend the combined oral contraceptive pill, even if you're not sexually active. This combined pill can often help improve acne in women, but may take up to a year before the full benefits are seen.

Co-cyprindiol

Co-cyprindiol is a hormonal treatment that can be used for more severe acne that doesn't respond to antibiotics. It helps to reduce the production of sebum.

You'll probably have to use co-cyprindiol for 2 to 6 months before you notice a significant improvement in your acne.

There's a small risk that women taking co-cyprindiol may develop breast cancer in later life.

For example, out of a group of 10,000 women who haven't taken co-cyprindiol, you would expect 16 of them to develop breast cancer by the time they were 35. This figure rises to 17 or 18 for women who were treated with co-cyprindiol for at least 5 years in their early twenties.

There's also a very small chance of co-cyprindiol causing a blood clot. The risk is estimated to be around 1 in 2,500 in any given year.

It's not thought to be safe to take co-cyprindiol if you're pregnant or breastfeeding. Women may need to have a pregnancy test before treatment can begin.

Other side effects of co-cyprindiol include:

• bleeding and spotting between your periods, which can sometimes occur for the first few months

• headaches

• sore breasts

• mood changes

• loss of interest in sex

• weight gain or weight loss

Isotretinoin

Isotretinoin has a number of beneficial effects:

• it helps to normalise sebum and reduce how much is produced

• it helps to prevent follicles becoming clogged

• it decreases the amount of bacteria on the skin

• it reduces redness and swelling in and around spots

However, the drug can also cause a wide range of side effects. It's only recommended for severe cases of acne that haven't responded to other treatments.

Because of the risk of side effects, isotretinoin can only be prescribed by a specially trained GP or a dermatologist.

Isotretinoin is taken as a tablet. Most people take a 4 to 6 month course. Your acne may get worse during the first 7 to 10 days of treatment. However, this is normal and soon settles.

Common side effects of isotretinoin include:

• inflammation, dryness and cracking of the skin, lips and nostrils

• changes in your blood sugar levels

• inflammation of your eyelids (blepharitis)

• inflammation and irritation of your eyes (conjunctivitis)

• blood in your urine

Rarer side effects of isotretinoin include:

• inflammation of the liver (hepatitis)

• inflammation of the pancreas (pancreatitis)

• kidney disease

Because of the risk of these rarer side effects, you'll need a blood test before and during treatment.

Isotretinoin and birth defects

Isotretinoin will damage an unborn baby. If you're a woman of childbearing age:

• don't use isotretinoin if you're pregnant or you think you're pregnant

• use 1, or ideally 2, methods of contraception for 1 month before treatment begins, during treatment and for 1 month after treatment has finished

• have a pregnancy test before, during and after treatment

You'll be asked to sign a form confirming that you understand the risk of birth defects and are willing to use contraceptives to prevent this risk, even if you're not currently sexually active.

If you think you may have become pregnant when taking isotretinoin, contact your dermatologist immediately.

Isotretinoin is also not suitable if you're breastfeeding.

Isotretinoin and mood changes

There have been reports of people experiencing mood changes while taking isotretinoin. There's no evidence that these mood changes were the result of the medication.

However, as a precaution, contact your doctor immediately if you feel depressed or anxious, have feelings of aggression or suicidal thoughts.

Non-pharmaceutical treatments

Several treatments for acne don't involve medication.

These include:

• comedone extractor – a small pen-shaped instrument that can be used to clean out blackheads and whiteheads

• chemical peels – where a chemical solution is applied to the face, causing the skin to peel off and new skin to replace it

• photodynamic therapy – where light is applied to the skin in an attempt to improve symptoms of acne

However, these treatments may not work and can't be routinely recommended.

Complications of acne

Acne scarring can sometimes develop as a complication of acne. Any type of acne spot can lead to scarring, but it's more common when the most serious types of spots (nodules and cysts) burst and damage nearby skin.

Scarring can also occur if you pick or squeeze your spots, so it's important not to do this.

There are 3 main types of acne scars:

• ice pick scars – small, deep holes in the surface of your skin that look like the skin has been punctured with a sharp object

• rolling scars – caused by bands of scar tissue that form under the skin, giving the surface of the skin a rolling and uneven appearance

• boxcar scars – round or oval depressions, or craters, in the skin

Treating acne scarring

Treatments for acne scarring are regarded as a type of cosmetic surgery, which isn't usually available on the NHS. However, in the past, exceptions have been made when it's been shown that acne scarring has caused serious psychological distress.

See your GP if you're considering having cosmetic surgery. They'll be able to discuss your options with you and advise you about the likelihood of having the procedure carried out on the NHS.

Many private clinics offer treatment for acne scarring. Prices can vary widely (from £500 to more than £10,000) depending on the type of treatment needed.

The British Association of Plastic, Reconstructive and Aesthetic Surgeons website has more information about private treatment available in your area.

It's important to have realistic expectations about what cosmetic treatment can achieve. While treatment can certainly improve the appearance of your scars, it can't get rid of them completely.

After treatment for acne scarring, most people notice a 50-75% improvement in their appearance.

Some of the available treatments for acne scarring are explained below.

Dermabrasion

Dermabrasion involves removing the top layer of skin, either using lasers or a specially made wire brush.

After the procedure, your skin will look red and sore for several months, but as it heals you should notice an improvement in the appearance of your scars.

Laser treatment

Laser treatment can be used to treat mild to moderate acne scarring. There are 2 types of laser treatment:

• ablative laser treatment – where lasers are used to remove a small patch of skin around the scar to produce a new, smooth-looking area of skin

• non-ablative laser treatment – where lasers are used to stimulate the growth of new collagen (a type of protein found in skin), which helps to repair some of the damage caused by scarring, and improves the appearance

Punch techniques

Punch techniques are used to treat ice pick scars and boxcar scars. There are 3 types of punch technique:

• punch excision – used to treat mild ice pick scars. The scar is surgically removed and the remaining wound is sealed. After the wound heals, it leaves a smoother and more even area of skin.

• punch elevation – used to treat boxcar scars. The base of the scar is surgically removed, leaving the sides of the scar in place. The base is then reattached to the sides, but lifted up so it's level with the surface of the skin. This makes the scar much less noticeable.

• punch grafting – used to treat very deep ice pick scars. As with a punch excision, the scar is removed, but the wound is "plugged" with a sample of skin taken from elsewhere on the body (usually from the back of the ear).

Subcision

Subcision is a surgical treatment that can be used to treat rolling scars. During surgery, the upper layer of the skin is removed from the underlying scar tissue. This allows blood to pool under the affected area. The blood clot helps form connective tissue, which pushes up the rolling scar so it's level with the rest of the surface of the skin.

Once subscision has been completed, additional treatment, such as laser treatment and dermabrasion, can be used to further improve the appearance of the scar.

Depression

Acne can often cause intense feelings of anxiety and stress, which can sometimes make people with the condition become socially withdrawn. This combination of factors can lead to people with acne becoming depressed.

You may be depressed if during the last month you've often felt down, depressed or hopeless, and have little interest or pleasure in doing things.

If you think that you or your child may have depression, it's important to speak to your GP.

Treatments for depression include:

• talking therapies such as cognitive behavioural therapy (CBT)

• a type of antidepressant called selective serotonin reuptake inhibitors (SSRIs)

9 798320 450247